Wood pellet smoker and grill cookbook

the ultimate guide for beginners and advanced users to barbecue and grill

Patrick sipperly

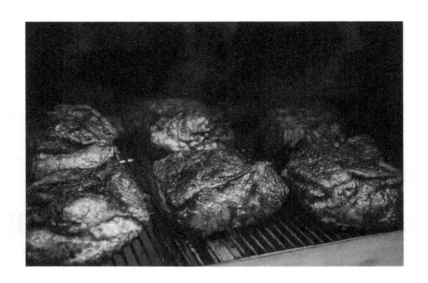

table of contents

The information in the following pages is broadly considered a truthful and accurate account of facts and as such, any inattention, use, or misuse of the information in question by the reader will render any resulting actions solely under their purview. There are no scenarios in which the publisher or the original author of this work can be in any fashion deemed liable for any hardship or damages that may befall them after undertaking information described herein.

Additionally, the information in the following pages is intended only for informational purposes and should thus be thought of as universal. As befitting its nature, it is presented without assurance regarding its prolonged validity or interim quality. Trademarks that are mentioned are done without written consent and can in no way be considered an endorsement from the trademark holder.

Introduction

The Fundamentals of Wood Pellet Smoking

Choosing Smoker

The significant and foremost step is to choose a smoker. You can invest in any type of smoker: charcoal smoker, gas smoker, or an electric smoker. A charcoal smoker runs for a long time and maintain steadier heat in the smoker and give pure meat flavors. A right choice for beginner cooks for smoking meat is a gas smoker where there is no need to monitor temperature, but it comes with a downside that meat won't have much flavor compared to charcoal. On the other hand, the most straightforward, most comfortable, and famous smoker is an electric smoker. Cooking with an electric smoker involves only two-step: turn it on, put meat in it, and walk away.

Choosing Fuel

Therefore, wood chips add a unique flavor to the meat and select that wood chips to enhance meat's taste. Some wood chips have a stronger flavor; some have mild while others are just enough to be alone for smoking. Check out the segment titled "types of smoker wood" to get to know and decide on wood chips that will complement your meat.

Type of Smoking Method

You have two choices to smoke meat, either using wet smoking, dry smoking, liquid smoke, or water smoking. Read the part "The core difference between cold and hot smoking" to determine the differences between each. Besides, go through the smoking meat portion in the unit, "the difference between barbecuing meat and smoking it."

Soaking Chips of Wood

Wood chips need to soak to the last longer for fueling smoking. The reason is dry wood that burns quickly, which means adding fuel to the smoker, resulting in dry smoked meat. There isn't any need to use wood chips when smoking for a shorter time. Prepare wood chips by soaking them in water for at least 4 hours before starting smoking. Then drain chips and wrap and seal them in an aluminum foil. Use a toothpick or fork for poking holes into the wood chips bag.

Set Smoker

Each type of smoker has its way of starting smoking. First, for wood or charcoal smoker, light up half of the charcoals and wait until their flame goes down. Then add remaining charcoal and wood chips if using. Wait, they are lighted and giving heat completely, then push charcoal aside and place the meat on the other side of the grilling grate. It is done to make sure that beef is indirectly smoked over low heat. Continue adding charcoal and soaked wood chips into the smoker.

For gas/propane or electric smoker, just turn it on according to manufacturer guideline and then add soaked wood chips into chip holder and fill water receptacle if a smoker has one. Either make use of the incorporated thermostat or buy your own to monitor the smoker's internal temperature. When the smoker reaches to desired preheated temperature, add meat to it.

Selecting Meat for Smoking

Choose the type of meat that tastes good with a smoky flavor. Following meat goes well for smoking.

- Beef: ribs, brisket, and corned beef.
- Pork: spare ribs, roast, shoulder, and ham.
- Poultry: whole chicken, a whole turkey, and big game hens.
- Seafood: Salmon, scallops, trout, and lobster

Getting Meat Ready

Prepare meat according to the recipe. Sometimes meat is cured, marinated, or simply seasoned with the rub. These preparation methods ensure smoked meat turns out flavorful, tender, and incredibly juicy.

Brine is a solution to treating poultry, pork, or ham. It involves dissolving brine ingredients in water poured into an enormous container and then adding meat. Then let soak for at minimum 8 hours and after that, rinse it well and pat dry before you begin smoking.

Marinate treat beef or briskets and add flavors to it. It's better to make deep cuts in meat to let marinate ingredients deep into it. Drain meat or smoke it straightaway.

Rubs are commonly used to treat beef, poultry, or ribs. They are a combination of salt and many spices, rubbed generously all over the meat. Then the meat is left to rest for at least 2 hours or more before smoking it.

Before smoking meat, make sure it is at room temperature. It ensures the meat is cooked evenly and reaches its internal temperature at the end of smoking time.

Beef Recipes

1. Grill a Burger Without Flipping Them

Preparation Time: 15 Minutes
Cooking Time: 50 Minutes
Servings: 6
Ingredients:

- 1 Ground Beef Patties

- Beef Rub

- Cheese
- Pretzel buns

Directions:

1. Start with cold but not frozen patties and sprinkle on the Beef Rub, and massage into both sides of the patty.

2. Preheat grill to 250 degrees and cook for 45 minutes

3. Add cheese and other topic varieties of your liking

4. Close the grill back up and let them finish for another 10 minutes before removing

Nutrition:

- Calories: 696 Cal
- Fat: 54 g
- Carbohydrates: 11 g
- Protein: 38 g

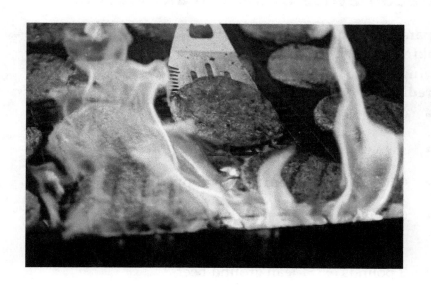

2. Bacon-Swiss Cheesesteak Meatloaf

Preparation Time: 15 Minutes
Cooking Time: 2 Hours
Servings: 8
Ingredients:

- One tablespoon canola oil

- Two garlic cloves, finely chopped

- One medium onion, finely chopped

- One poblano chile stemmed, seeded, and finely chopped

- 2 pounds extra-lean ground beef

- Two tablespoons Montreal steak seasoning

- One tablespoon A.1. Steak Sauce

- ½ pound bacon, cooked and crumbled

- 2 cups shredded Swiss cheese

- One egg, beaten

- 2 cups breadcrumbs

- ½ cup Tiger Sauce

Directions:

1. On your stovetop, heat the canola oil in a medium sauté pan over medium-high heat.

2. Add the garlic, onion, and poblano, and sauté for 3 to 5 minutes, or until the onion is just barely translucent.

3. Supply your smoker with wood pellets.

4. Preheat, with the lid closed, to 225°F.

5. In a large bowl, combine the sautéed vegetables, ground beef, steak seasoning, steak sauce, bacon, Swiss cheese, egg, and breadcrumbs.

6. Mix with your hands until well incorporated, then shape into a loaf.

7. Put the meatloaf in a cast-iron skillet and place it on the grill.

8. Insert meat thermometer inserted in the loaf reads 165°F.

9. Top with the meatloaf with the Tiger Sauce, remove from the grill and rest for about 10 minutes before serving.

Nutrition:
- Calories: 120 Cal
- Fat: 2 g
- Carbohydrates: 0 g
- Protein: 23 g

3. London Broil

Preparation Time: 20 Minutes
Cooking Time: 16 Minutes
Servings: 4
Ingredients:

- 1 (1½- to 2-pound) London broil or top round steak

- ¼ cup of soy sauce

- Two tablespoons white wine

- Two tablespoons extra-virgin olive oil

- ¼ cup chopped scallions

- Two tablespoons packed brown sugar

- Two garlic cloves, minced

- Two teaspoons red pepper flakes

- One teaspoon freshly ground black pepper

Directions:

1. Using a meat mallet, pound the steak lightly all over on both sides to break down its fibers and tenderize. You are not trying to pound down the thickness.

2. In a medium bowl, make the marinade by combining the soy sauce, white wine, olive oil, scallions, brown sugar, garlic, red pepper flakes, and black pepper.

3. Put the steak in a shallow plastic container with a lid and pour the marinade over the meat. Cover and refrigerate for 4 hours.

4. Stock your smoker with wood pellets and follow the manufacturer's specific start-up guidelines.

5. Preheat, with the lid shut, to 350°F.

6. Place the steak directly on the grill, close the lid, and smoke for 6 minutes.

7. Flip, then smoke with the lid closed for 6 to 10 minutes more, or until a meat thermometer inserted in the meat reads 130°F for medium-rare.

8. The meat's temperature will rise by about 5 degrees while it rests.

Nutrition:
- Calories: 316 Cal
- Fat: 3 g
- Carbohydrates: 0 g
- Protein: 54 g

4. Beef Shoulder Clod

Preparation Time: 10 Minutes
Cooking Time: 16 Hours
Servings: 20
Ingredients:

- ½ cup of sea salt

- ½ cup freshly ground black pepper

- One tablespoon red pepper flake

- One tablespoon minced garlic

- One tablespoon cayenne pepper

- One tablespoon smoked paprika

- 1 (13- to 15-pound) beef shoulder clod

Directions:

1. Combine spices

2. Generously apply it to the beef shoulder.

3. Supply your smoker with wood pellets and trail the manufacturer's specific start-up guidelines.

4. Preheat, with the lid locked, to 250°F.

5. Put the meat on the grill grate, close the lid, smoke for 12 to 16 hours, or until a meat thermometer inserted deeply into the beef reads 195°F.

6. You may need to cover the clod with aluminum foil toward the end of smoking to prevent over-browning.

7. Let the meat rest and serve

Nutrition:

- Calories: 290 Cal
- Fat: 22 g
- Carbohydrates: 0 g
- Protein: 20 g

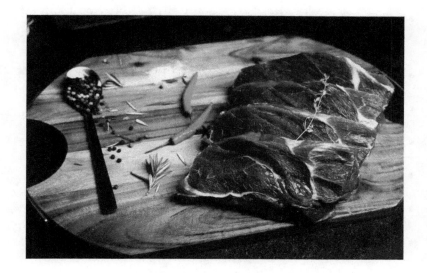

5. Corned Beef and Cabbage

Preparation Time: 30 Minutes
Cooking Time: 5 Hours
Servings: 8
Ingredients:

- 1-gallon water

- 1 (3- to 4-pound) pointcut corned beef brisket with pickling spice packet

- One tablespoon freshly ground black pepper

- One tablespoon garlic powder

- ½ cup molasses

- One teaspoon ground mustard

- One head green cabbage

- Four tablespoons (½ stick) butter

- Two tablespoons rendered bacon fat

- One chicken bouillon cube, crushed

Directions:

1. turning the spray as regularly as you remember, every 3 hours while you're awake – to wash out some as you look back to do so – ideally, every 3 hours while you're awake – to soak out some of the curing salt initially added.

2. Supply your smoker with wood pellets and tail the manufacturer's specific start-up procedure.

3. Preheat to 275°F.

4. Remove the meat from the brining liquid, pat it dry, and generously rub with the black pepper and garlic powder.

5. Put the seasoned corned beef directly on the grill, fat-side up, close the lid, and grill for 2 hours.

6. Remove from the grill when done.

7. In a bowl, combine the molasses and ground mustard and pour half of this mixture into the bottom of a disposable aluminum pan.

8. Transfer the meat to the pan, fat-side up, and pour the remaining molasses mixture on top, spreading it evenly over the meat.

9. Cover tightly with aluminum foil.

10. Transfer the pan to the grill, close the lid, and continue smoking the corned beef for 2 to 3 hours or until a meat thermometer inserted in the thickest part reads 185°F.

11. Rest meat

12. Serve.

Nutrition:
- Calories: 295 Cal
- Fat: 17 g
- Carbohydrates: 19 g
- Protein: 18 g
- Fiber: 6 g

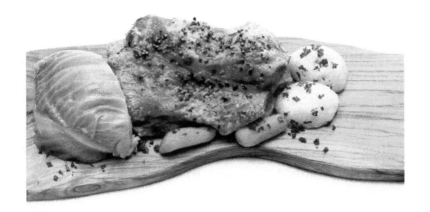

6. Cheeseburger Hand Pies

Preparation Time: 35 Minutes
Cooking Time: 10 Minutes
Servings: 6
Ingredients:

- ½ pound lean ground beef

- One tablespoon minced onion

- One tablespoon steak seasoning

- 1 cup cheese

- Eight slices of white American cheese, divided

- 2 (14-ounce) refrigerated prepared pizza dough sheets, divided

- Two eggs

- 24 hamburger dill pickle chips

- Two tablespoons sesame seeds

- Six slices tomato, for garnish

- Ketchup and mustard, for serving

Directions:

1. Supply your smoker thru wood pellets and follow the manufacturer's specific start-up.

2. Preheat, with the lid closed, to 325°F.

3. On your stovetop, in a medium sauté pan over medium-high heat, brown the ground beef for 4 to 5 minutes, or until cooked through.

4. Add the minced onion and steak seasoning.

5. Toss in the shredded cheese blend and two slices of American cheese and stir until melted and fully incorporated.

6. Remove the cheeseburger mixture from the heat and set aside.

7. Make sure the dough is well chilled for easier handling.

8. Working quickly, roll out one prepared pizza crust on parchment paper and brush with half of the egg wash.

9. Arrange the remaining six slices of American cheese on the dough to outline six hand pies.

Nutrition:
- Calories: 325 Cal
- Fat: 21 g
- Carbohydrates: 11 g
- Protein: 23 g

7. Pastrami

Preparation Time: 10 Minutes
Cooking Time: 5 Hours
Servings: 12
Ingredients:

- 1-gallon water, plus ½ cup

- ½ cup packed light brown sugar

- 1 (3- to 4-pound) pointcut corned beef brisket with brine mix packet

- Two tablespoons freshly ground black pepper

- ¼ cup ground coriander

Directions:

1. Cover and refrigerate overnight, changing the water as often as you remember to do so — ideally, every 3 hours while you're awake — to wash out some of the curing salt initially added.

2. Supply your smoker with wood pellets and trail the manufacturer's specific start-up.

3. Heat up, with the lid closed, to 275°F.

4. In a small bowl, combine the black pepper and ground coriander to form a rub.

5. Drain the meat, pat it dry, and generously coat on all sides with the rub.

6. Place the corned beef directly on the grill, fat-side up, close the lid, and smoke for 3 hours to 3 hours 30

minutes, or until a meat thermometer inserted in the thickest part reads 175°F to 185°F.

7. Add the corned beef, cover tightly with aluminum foil, and smoke on the grill with the lid closed for an additional 30 minutes to 1 hour.

8. Remove the meat

9. Refrigerate

Nutrition:

- Calories: 123 Cal
- Fat: 4 g
- Carbohydrates: 3 g
- Protein: 16 g
- Fiber: 0 g

8. Traeger Beef Jerky

Preparation Time: 15 Minutes
Cooking Time: 5 Hours
Servings: 10
Ingredients:

- 3 pounds sirloin steaks

- 2 cups soy sauce

- 1 cup pineapple juice

- 1/2 cup brown sugar

- 2 tbsp sriracha

- 2 tbsp hoisin

- 2 tbsp red pepper flake

- 2 tbsp rice wine vinegar

- 2 tbsp onion powder

Directions:

1. Mix the flavoring in a zip lock bag, then add the beef.

2. Mix until well coated and remove as much air as possible.

3. Place the bag in a fridge and let marinate overnight or for 6 hours.

4. Remove the bag from the fridge an hour before cooking

5. Startup the Traeger and set it on the smoking settings or at 1900F.

6. Lay the meat on the grill leaving a half-inch space between the pieces.

7. Let cool for 5 hours and turn after 2 hours.

8. Remove from the grill and let cool. Serve or refrigerate

Nutrition:
- Calories: 309 Cal
- Fat: 7 g
- Carbohydrates: 20 g
- Protein: 34 g
- Fiber: 1 g

9. Traeger Smoked Beef Roast

Preparation Time: 10 Minutes
Cooking Time: 6 Hours
Servings: 6
Ingredients:

- 1-3/4 pounds beef sirloin tip

- 1/2 cup barbeque rub

- Two bottles of amber beer

- One bottle BBQ sauce

Directions:

1. Turn the Traeger onto the smoke setting.

2. Rub the beef with barbeque rub until well coated, then place on the grill.

3. Let smoke for 4 hours while flipping every 1 hour.

4. Transfer the beef to a pan and add the beer. The meat should be 1/2 way covered.

5. Braise the beef until fork tender. It will take 3 hours on the stovetop and 60 minutes on the instant pot.

6. Remove the beef from the ban and reserve 1 cup of the cooking liquid.

7. Use two forks to shred the beef into small pieces, then return to the pan with the reserved braising liquid. Add BBQ sauce and stir well, then keep warm until serving. You can also reheat if it gets cold.

Nutrition:

- Calories: 829 Cal
- Fat: 18 g
- Carbohydrates: 4 g
- Protein: 86 g

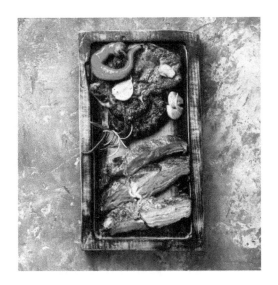

10. Reverse Seared Flank Steak

Preparation Time: 10 Minutes
Cooking Time: 20 Minutes
Servings: 2
Ingredients:

- 3-pound flank steaks

- 1 tbsp salt

- 1/2 tbsp onion powder

- 1/4 tbsp garlic powder

- 1/2 black pepper, coarsely ground

Directions:

1. Preheat the Traeger to 2250F.

2. Add the steaks and rub them generously with the rub mixture.

3. Place the steak

4. Let cook until its internal temperature is 100F under your desired temperature. 1150F for rare, 1250F for the medium rear, and 1350F for medium.

5. Wrap the steak with foil and raise the grill temperature to high.

6. Place back the steak and grill for 3 minutes on each side.

7. Pat with butter and serve when hot.

Nutrition:

- Calories: 112 Cal
- Fat: 5 g
- Carbohydrates: 1 g
- Protein: 16 g
- Fiber: 0 g

11. Traeger New York Strip

Preparation Time: 5 Minutes
Cooking Time: 15 Minutes
Servings: 6
Ingredients:

- 3 New York strips

- Salt and pepper

Directions:

1. If the steak is in the fridge, remove it 30 minutes before cooking.

2. Preheat the Traeger to 4500F.

3. Meanwhile, season the steak generously with salt and pepper.

4. Place it on the grill and let it cook for 5 minutes per side or until the internal temperature reaches 1280F.

5. Rest for 10 minutes.

Nutrition:

- Calories: 198 Cal
- Fat: 14 g
- Carbohydrates: 0 g
- Protein: 17 g

Pork Recipes

12. Simple Wood Pellet Smoked Pork Ribs

Preparation Time: 15 Minutes
Cooking Time: 5 Hours
Servings: 7
Ingredients:

- Three rack baby back ribs

- 3/4 cup pork and poultry rub

- 3/4 cup Que BBQ Sauce

Directions:

1. Peel the membrane from the backside of the ribs and trim any fat.

2. Season the pork generously with the rub.

3. Set the wood pellet grill to 180°F and preheat for 15 minutes with the lid closed.

4. Place the pork ribs on the grill and smoke them for 5 hours.

5. Remove it from the grill and wrap them in a foil with the BBQ sauce.

6. Place back the pork and increase the temperature to 350°F — Cook for 45 more minutes.

7. Remove the pork from the grill and let it rest for 20 minutes before serving. Enjoy.

Nutrition:

- Calories 762
- Total Fat 57g
- Saturated Fat 17g
- Total Carbs 23g
- Net Carbs 22.7g
- Protein 39g
- Sugar 18g
- Fiber 0.5g
- Sodium: 737mg
- Potassium 618mg

13. Roasted Pork with Balsamic Strawberry Sauce

Preparation Time: 15 Minutes
Cooking Time: 35 Minutes
Servings: 3
Ingredients:

- 2 lb. pork tenderloin

- Salt and pepper to taste

- 2 tbsp rosemary, dried

- 2 tbsp olive oil

- 12 strawberries, fresh

- 1 cup balsamic vinegar

- 4 tbsp sugar

Directions:

1. Set the wood pellet grill to 350°F and preheat for 15 minutes with a closed lid.

2. Meanwhile, rinse the pork and pat it dry — season with salt, pepper, and rosemary.

3. In an oven skillet, heat oil until smoking. Add the pork and sear on all sides until golden brown.

4. Set the skillet in the grill and cook for 20 minutes or until the meat is no longer pink and the internal temperature is 150°F.

5. Remove the pork from the grill and let rest for 10 minutes.

6. Add berries to the skillet and sear over the stovetop for a minute. Remove the strawberries from the skillet.

7. Add vinegar in the same skillet and scrape any browned bits from the skillet bottom. Bring it to boil, then reduce heat to low. Stir in sugar and cook until it has reduced by half.

8. Slice the meat and place the strawberries on top, then drizzle vinegar sauce. Enjoy.

Nutrition:
- Calories 244
- Total Fat 9g
- Saturated Fat 3g
- Total Carbs 15g
- Net Carbs 13g
- Protein 25g
- Sugar 12g
- Fiber 2g
- Sodium: 159mg

14. Wood Pellet Grill Pork Crown Roast

Preparation Time: 5 Minutes
Cooking Time: 60 Minutes
Servings: 5
Ingredients:

- 13 ribs pork

- 1/4 cup favorite rub

- 1 cup apple juice

- 1 cup Apricot BBQ sauce

Directions:

1. Set the wood pellet temperature to 375°F to preheat for 15 minutes with the lid closed.

2. Meanwhile, season the pork with the rub, then let sit for 30 minutes.

3. Wrap the tips of each crown roast with foil to prevent the burns from turning black.

4. Place the meat on the grill grate and cook for 90 minutes. Spray apple juice every 30 minutes.

5. When the meat has reached an internal temperature of 125°F, remove the foils.

6. Spray the roast with apple juice again and let cook until the internal temperature has reached 135°F.

7. In the latter 10 minutes of cooking, baste the roast with BBQ sauce.

8. Remove from the grill and wrap with foil. Let rest for 15 minutes before serving. Enjoy.

Nutrition:

- Calories 240
- Total fat 16g
- Saturated fat 6g
- Protein 23g
- Sodium: 50mg

15. Wet-Rubbed St. Louis Ribs

Preparation Time: 15 Minutes
Cooking Time: 4 Hours
Servings: 3
Ingredients:

- 1/2 cup brown sugar

- 1 tbsp cumin, ground

- 1 tbsp Ancho Chile powder

- 1 tbsp smoked paprika

- 1 tbsp garlic salt

- 3 tbsp balsamic vinegar

- 1 Rack St. Louis style ribs

- 2 cup apple juice

Directions:

1. Add all the ingredients except ribs in a mixing bowl and mix until well mixed. Place the rub on both sides of the ribs and let sit for 10 minutes.

2. Set the wood pellet temperature to 180°F and preheat for 15 minutes. Smoke the ribs for 2 hours.

3. Increase the temperature to 250°F and wrap the ribs and apple juice with foil or tinfoil.

4. Place back the pork and cook for an additional 2 hours.

5. Remove from the grill and let rest for 5 minutes before serving. Enjoy.

Nutrition:

- Calories 210
- Total fat 13g
- Saturated fat 4g
- Total Carbs 0g
- Net Carbs 0g
- Protein 24g
- Sodium: 85mg

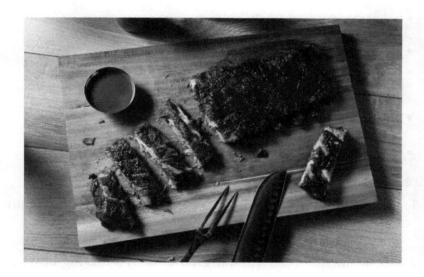

16. Cocoa Crusted Pork Tenderloin

Preparation Time: 30 Minutes
Cooking Time: 25 Minutes
Servings: 5
Ingredients:

- One pork tenderloin

- 1/2 tbsp fennel, ground

- 2 tbsp cocoa powder, unsweetened

- 1 tbsp smoked paprika

- 1/2 tbsp kosher salt

- 1/2 tbsp black pepper

- 1 tbsp extra virgin olive oil

- Three green onion

Directions:

1. Remove the silver skin and the connective tissues from the pork loin.

2. Combine the rest of the ingredients in a mixing bowl, then rub the mixture on the pork. Refrigerate for 30 minutes.

3. Preheat the wood pellet grill for 15 minutes with the lid closed.

4. Sear all sides of the loin at the front of the grill, then reduce the temperature to 350°F and move the pork to the center grill.

5. Cook for 15 more minutes or until the internal temperature is 145°F.

6. Remove from grill and let rest for 10 minutes before slicing. Enjoy

Nutrition:

- Calories 264
- Total fat 13.1g
- Saturated fat 6g
- Total Carbs 4.6g
- Net Carbs 1.2g
- Protein 33g
- Sugar 0g
- Fiber 3.4g
- Sodium: 66mg

17. Wood Pellet Grilled Bacon

Preparation Time: 30 Minutes
Cooking Time: 25 Minutes
Servings: 6
Ingredients:

- 1 lb. bacon, thickly cut

Directions:

1. Preheat your wood pellet grill to 375°F.

2. Line a baking sheet with parchment paper, then place the bacon on it in a single layer.

3. Close the lid and bake for 20 minutes. Flip over, close the top, and bake for an additional 5 minutes.

4. Serve with the favorite side and enjoy it.

Nutrition:

- Calories 315
- Total fat 14g
- Saturated fat 10g
- Protein 9g
- Sodium: 500mg

18. Wood Pellet Grilled Pork Chops

Preparation Time: 20 Minutes
Cooking Time: 10 Minutes
Servings: 6
Ingredients:

- Six pork chops, thickly cut

- BBQ rub

Directions:

1. Preheat the wood pellet to 450°F.

2. Season the pork chops generously with the BBQ rub. Place the pork chops on the grill and cook for 6 minutes or until the internal temperature reaches 145°F.

3. Remove from the grill and let sit for 10 minutes before serving.

4. Enjoy.

Nutrition:

- Calories 264
- Total fat 13g
- Saturated fat 6g
- Total Carbs 4g
- Net Carbs 1g
- Protein 33g
- Fiber 3g
- Sodium: 66mg

19. Wood Pellet Blackened Pork Chops

Preparation Time: 5 Minutes
Cooking Time: 20 Minutes
Servings: 6
Ingredients:

- Six pork chops

- 1/4 cup blackening seasoning

- Salt and pepper to taste

Directions:

1. Preheat your grill to 375°F.

2. Meanwhile, generously season the pork chops with the blackening seasoning, salt, and pepper.

3. Place the pork chops on the grill and close the lid.

4. Let grill for 8 minutes, then flip the chops. Cook until the internal temperature reaches 142°F.

5. Remove the chops from the grill and let rest for 10 minutes before slicing.

6. Serve and enjoy.

Nutrition:

- Calories 333
- Total fat 18g
- Saturated fat 6g
- Total Carbs 1g
- Protein 40g,
- Fiber 1g
- Sodium: 3175mg

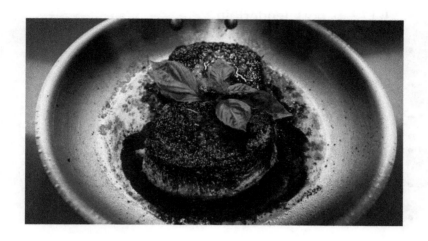

20. Teriyaki Pineapple Pork Tenderloin Sliders

Preparation Time: 20 Minutes
Cooking Time: 20 Minutes

Servings: 6
Ingredients:

- 1-1/2 lb. pork tenderloin

- One can pineapple ring

- One package king's Hawaiian rolls

- 8 oz teriyaki sauce

- 1-1/2 tbsp salt

- 1 tbsp onion powder

- 1 tbsp paprika

- 1/2 tbsp garlic powder

- 1/2 tbsp cayenne pepper

Directions:

1. Add all the fixings for the rub in a mixing bowl and mix until well mixed. Generously rub the pork loin with the mixture.

2. Heat the pellet to 325°F. Place the meat on a grill and cook while you turn it every 4 minutes.

3. Cook until the internal temperature reaches 145°F.remove from the grill and let it rest for 5 minutes.

4. Meanwhile, open the pineapple can and place the pineapple rings on the grill. Flip the rings when they have a dark brown color.

5. At the same time, half the rolls and place them on the grill and grill them until toasty browned.

6. Assemble the slider by putting the bottom roll first, followed by the pork tenderloin, pineapple ring, a drizzle of sauce, and top with the other roll half. Serve and enjoy.

Nutrition:

- Calories 243
- Total fat 5g
- Saturated fat 2g
- Total Carbs 4g
- Net Carbs 15g
- Protein 33g
- Sugar 10g,
- Fiber 1g
- Sodium: 2447mg

21. Wood Pellet Grilled Tenderloin with Fresh Herb Sauce

Preparation Time: 10 Minutes
Cooking Time: 15 Minutes
Servings: 4
Ingredients:

- One pork tenderloin, silver skin removed and dried

- BBQ seasoning

- One handful basil, fresh

- 1/4 tbsp garlic powder

- 1/3 cup olive oil

- 1/2 tbsp kosher salt

Directions:

1. Preheat the wood pellet grill to medium heat.

2. Coat the pork with BBQ seasoning, then cook on semi-direct heat of the grill. Turn the pork regularly to ensure even cooking.

3. Cook until the internal temperature is 145°F. Remove from the grill and let it rest for 10 minutes.

4. Meanwhile, make the herb sauce by pulsing all the sauce ingredients in a food processor — pulse for a few times or until well chopped.

5. Slice the pork diagonally and spoon the sauce on top. Serve and enjoy.

Nutrition:

- Calories 300
- Total fat 22g
- Saturated fat 4g
- Total Carbs 13g
- Net Carbs 12g
- Protein 14g
- Sugar 10g
- Fiber 1g
- Sodium: 791mg

22. Wood Pellet Grilled Shredded Pork Tacos

Preparation Time: 15 Minutes
Cooking Time: 7 Hours
Servings: 8
Ingredients:

- 5 lb. pork shoulder, bone-in

- 3 tbsp brown sugar

- 1 tbsp salt

- 1 tbsp garlic powder

- 1 tbsp paprika

- 1 tbsp onion powder

- 1/4 tbsp cumin

- 1 tbsp cayenne pepper

Directions:

1. Mix all the dry rub ingredients and rub on the pork shoulder.

2. Preheat the grill to 275°F and cook the pork directly for 6 hours or until the internal temperature has reached 145°F.

3. If you want to fall off the bone tender pork, then cook until the internal temperature is 190°F.

4. Let rest for 10 minutes before serving. Enjoy

Nutrition:

- Calories 566

- Total fat 41g
- Saturated fat 15g
- Total Carbs 4g
- Net Carbs 4g
- Protein 44g
- Sugar 3g
- Fiber 0g
- Sodium: 659mg

23. Wood Pellet Togarashi Pork Tenderloin

Preparation Time: 5 Minutes
Cooking Time: 25 Minutes
Servings: 6
Ingredients:

- 1 Pork tenderloin

- 1/2tbsp kosher salt

- 1/4 cup Togarashi seasoning

Directions:

1. Cut any excess silver skin from the pork and sprinkle with salt to taste. Rub generously with the togarashi seasoning

2. Place in a preheated oven at 400°F for 25 minutes or until the internal temperature reaches 145°F.

3. Remove from the grill and let rest for 10 minutes before slicing and serving.

4. Enjoy.

Nutrition:

- Calories 390
- Total fat 13g
- Saturated fat 6g
- Total Carbs 4g
- Net Carbs 1g
- Protein 33g
- Sugar 0g
- Fiber 3g

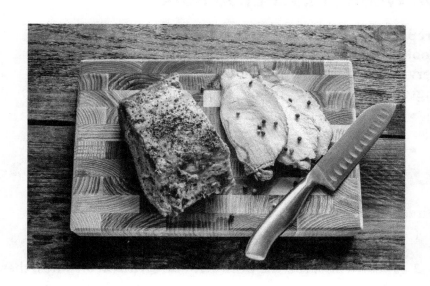

24. Wood Pellet Pulled Pork

Preparation Time: 15 Minutes
Cooking Time: 12 Hours
Servings: 12
Ingredients:

- 8 lb. pork shoulder roast, bone-in

- BBQ rub

- 3 cups apple cider, dry hard

Directions:

1. Fire up the wood pellet grill and set it to smoke.

2. Meanwhile, rub the pork with BBQ rub on all sides, then place it on the grill grates. Cook for 5 hours, flipping it every 1 hour.

3. Increase the heat to 225°F and continue cooking for 3 hours directly on the grate.

4. Transfer the pork to a foil pan and place the apple cider at the bottom of the pan.

5. Cook until the internal temperature reaches 200°F then remove it from the grill. Wrap the pork loosely with foil, then let it rest for 1 hour.

6. Remove the fat layer and use forks to shred it.

7. Serve and enjoy.

Nutrition:

- Calories 912
- Total fat 65g
- Saturated fat 24g

- Total Carbs 7g
- Net Carbs 7g
- Protein 70g
- Sugar 6g
- Fiber 0g
- Sodium: 208mg

Poultry Recipes

25. Buffalo Chicken Wings

Preparation Time: 15 Minutes
Cooking Time: 25 Minutes
Servings: 6
Ingredients:

- 2 lb. chicken wings

- 1/2 cup sweet, spicy dry rub

- 2/3 cup buffalo sauce

- Celery, chopped

Directions:

1. Start your wood pellet grill.

2. Set it to 450 degrees F.

3. Sprinkle the chicken wings with the dry rub.

4. Place on the grill rack.

5. Cook for 10 minutes per side.

6. Brush with the buffalo sauce.

7. Grill for another 5 minutes.

8. Dip each wing in the buffalo sauce.

9. Sprinkle the celery on top.

Nutrition:

- Calories 935

- Total fat 53g
- Saturated fat 15g
- Protein 107g
- Sodium 320mg

26. Sweet and Sour Chicken

Preparation Time: 30 Minutes
Cooking Time: 5 Hours
Servings: 4
Ingredients:

- Eight chicken drumsticks

- 1/4 cup soy sauce

- 1 cup ketchup

- Two tablespoons rice wine vinegar

- Two tablespoons lemon juice

- Two tablespoons honey

- Two tablespoons garlic, minced

- Two tablespoons ginger, minced

- One tablespoon sweet-spicy dry rub

- Three tablespoons brown sugar

Directions:

1. Combine all the sauce fixings in a bowl.

2. Mix well.

3. Take half of the mixture, transfer to another bowl and refrigerate.

4. Add the chicken to the bowl with the remaining sauce.

5. Toss to coat evenly.

6. Cover and refrigerate for 4 hours.

7. When ready to cook, take the chicken out of the refrigerator.

8. Discard the marinade.

9. Turn on your wood pellet grill.

10. Set it to smoke.

11. Set the temperature to 225 degrees F.

12. Smoke the chicken for 3 hours.

13. Serve the chicken with the reserved sauce.

Nutrition:
- Calories 935
- Total fat 53g
- Saturated fat 15g
- Protein 107g
- Sodium 320mg

27. Honey Glazed Whole Chicken

Preparation Time: 30 Minutes
Cooking Time: 4 Hours
Servings: 4
Ingredients:

- One tablespoon honey

- Four tablespoons butter

- Three tablespoons lemon juice

- One whole chicken, giblets trimmed

- Four tablespoons chicken seasoning

Directions:

1. Set your wood pellet grill to smoke.

2. Set it to 225 degrees F.

3. In a pan over low heat, increase the honey and butter. Pour in the lemon juice.

4. Add the seasoning.

5. Cook for 1 minute, stirring.

6. Add the chicken to the grill.

7. Smoke for 8 minutes.

8. Flip the chicken and brush with the honey mixture.

9. Smoke for 3 hours, brushing the sauce every 40 minutes.

10. Let rest for 5 minutes before serving.

Nutrition:

- Calories 935
- Total fat 53g
- Saturated fat 15g
- Protein 107g
- Sodium 320mg

28. Chicken Lollipops

Preparation Time: 30 Minutes
Cooking Time: 2 Hours
Servings: 6
Ingredients:

- 12 chicken lollipops

- Chicken seasoning

- Ten tablespoons butter, sliced into 12 cubes

- 1 cup barbecue sauce

- 1 cup hot sauce

Directions:

1. Turn on your wood pellet grill.

2. Set it to 300 degrees F.

3. Then season, the chicken with the chicken seasoning.

4. Arrange the chicken in a baking pan.

5. Put the butter cubes on top of each chicken.

6. Cook the chicken lollipops for 2 hours, basting with the melted butter in the baking pan every 20 minutes.

7. Pour in the barbecue sauce and hot sauce over the chicken.

8. Grill for 15 minutes.

Nutrition:

- Calories 935
- Total fat 53g

- Saturated fat 15g
- Protein 107g
- Sodium 320mg

29. Asian Wings

Preparation Time: 30 Minutes
Cooking Time: 3 Hours
Servings: 6
Ingredients:

- One teaspoon honey

- One teaspoon soy sauce

- Two teaspoon rice vinegar

- 1/2 cup hoisin sauce

- Two teaspoon sesame oil

- One teaspoon ginger, minced

- One teaspoon garlic, minced

- One teaspoon green onion, chopped

- 1 cup hot water

- 2 lb. chicken wings

Directions:

1. Combine all the sauce fixings in a large bowl. Mix well.

2. Transfer 1/3 of the sauce to another bowl and refrigerate.

3. Add the chicken wings to the remaining sauce.

4. Cover and refrigerate for 2 hours.

5. Turn on your wood pellet grill.

6. Set it to 300 degrees F.

7. Add the wings to a grilling basket.

8. Cook for 1 hour.

9. Heat the reserved sauce in a pan.

10. Bring to a boil and then simmer for 10 minutes.

11. Brush the chicken with the remaining sauce.

12. Grill for another 10 minutes.

13. Let rest for 5 minutes before serving.

Nutrition:
- Calories 935
- Total fat 53g
- Saturated fat 15g
- Protein 107g
- Sodium 320mg

30. Lemon Chicken in Foil Packet

Preparation Time: 5 Minutes
Cooking Time: 25 Minutes
Servings: 4
Ingredients:

- Four chicken fillets

- Three tablespoons melted butter

- One garlic, minced

- 1-1/2 teaspoon dried Italian seasoning

- Salt and pepper to taste

- One lemon, sliced

Directions:

1. Turn on your wood pellet grill.

2. Keep the lid open while burning for 5 minutes.

3. Preheat it to 450 degrees F.

4. Add the chicken fillet on top of foil sheets.

5. In a bowl, mix the butter, garlic, seasoning, salt, and pepper.

6. Brush the chicken with this mixture.

7. Put the lemon slices on top.

8. Wrap the chicken with the foil.

9. Grill each side for 7 to 10 minutes per side.

Nutrition:

- Calories 935
- Total fat 53g
- Saturated fat 15g
- Protein 107g
- Sodium 320mg

31. Sweet and Spicy Chicken

Preparation Time: 30 Minutes
Cooking Time: 1 Hour and 30 Minutes
Servings: 4
Ingredients:

- 16 chicken wings

- Three tablespoons lime juice

- A sweet, spicy rub

Directions:

1. Arrange the chicken wings in a baking pan.

2. Pour the lime juice over the wings.

3. Sprinkle the wings with the seasoning.

4. Set your wood pellet grill to 350 degrees F.

5. Add the chicken wings to the grill.

6. Grill for 20 minutes per side.

Nutrition:

- Calories 935
- Total fat 53g
- Saturated fat 15g
- Protein 107g
- Sodium 320mg

32. Teriyaki Turkey

Preparation Time: 30 Minutes
Cooking Time: 4 Hours
Servings: 10
Ingredients:
Glaze

- 1/4 cup melted butter

- 1/2 cup apple cider

- Two cloves garlic, minced

- 1/2 teaspoon ground ginger

- Two tablespoons soy sauce

- Two tablespoons honey

Turkey

- Two tablespoons chicken seasoning

- One whole turkey

Thickener

- One tablespoon cold water

- One teaspoon cornstarch

Directions:

1. Add the glaze ingredients to a pan over medium heat.

2. Bring to a boil and then simmer for 5 minutes.

3. Reserve 5 tablespoons of the mixture.

4. Add the remaining to a marinade injection.

5. Place the turkey in a baking pan.

6. Season with the chicken seasoning.

7. Turn on the wood pellet grill.

8. Set it to 300 degrees F.

9. Add the turkey to the grill.

10. Cook for 3 hours.

11. Add the thickener to the reserved mixture.

12. Brush the turkey with this sauce.

13. Cook for another 1 hour.

Nutrition:

- Calories 935
- Total fat 53g
- Saturated fat 15g
- Protein 107g
- Sodium 320mg

33. Cheesy Turkey Burger

Preparation Time: 20 Minutes
Cooking Time: 3 Hours
Servings: 8
Ingredients:

- 3 lb. ground turkey

- Burger seasoning

- 7 oz. brie cheese, sliced into cubes

- Eight burger buns, sliced

- Blueberry jam

- Two roasted bell peppers, sliced

Directions:

1. Season the turkey with the burger seasoning.

2. Mix well.

3. Form 8 patties from the mixture.

4. Press cheese into the patties.

5. Cover the top with more turkey.

6. Preheat your wood pellet grill to 350 degrees F.

7. Cook the turkey burgers for 30 to 40 minutes per side.

8. Spread the burger buns with blueberry jam.

9. Add the turkey burger on top.

10. Top with the bell peppers.

Nutrition:

- Calories 935
- Total fat 53g
- Saturated fat 15g
- Protein 107g
- Sodium 320mg

34. Turkey Sandwich

Preparation Time: 5 Minutes
Cooking Time: 25 Minutes
Servings: 4
Ingredients:

- Eight bread slices

- 1 cup gravy

- 2 cups turkey, cooked and shredded

Directions:

1. Set your wood pellet grill to smoke.

2. Preheat it to 400 degrees F.

3. Place a grill mat on top of the grates.

4. Add the turkey on top of the mat.

5. Cook for 10 minutes.

6. Toast the bread in the flame broiler.

7. Top the bread with the gravy and shredded turkey.

Nutrition:

- Calories 935
- Total fat 53g
- Saturated fat 15g
- Protein 107g
- Sodium 320mg

35. Smoked Turkey

Preparation Time: 30 Minutes
Cooking Time: 6 Hours and 30 Minutes
Servings: 8
Ingredients:

- 1 cup butter

- 1/2 cup maple syrup

- Two tablespoons chicken seasoning

- One whole turkey

Directions:

1. Add the butter to a pan over low heat.

2. Stir in the maple syrup.

3. Simmer for 5 minutes, stirring.

4. Turn off the stove and let cool.

5. Add to a marinade injection.

6. Inject into the turkey.

7. Add the turkey to the wood pellet grill.

8. Set it smoke.

9. Smoke at 275 degrees F for 6 hours.

Nutrition:

- Calories 935
- Total fat 53g
- Saturated fat 15g
- Protein 107g

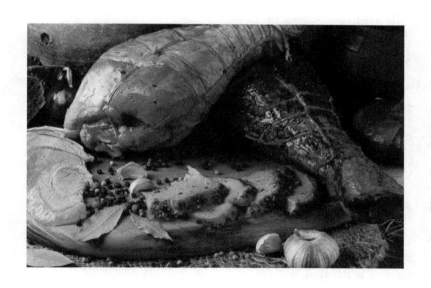

36. Texas Turkey

Preparation Time: 30 Minutes
Cooking Time: 4 Hours and 30 Minutes
Servings: 8
Ingredients:

- One pre-brined turkey

- Salt and pepper to taste

- 1 lb. butter

Directions:

1. Preheat your wood pellet grill to 300 degrees F.

2. Season the turkey with salt and pepper.

3. Grill for 3 hours.

4. Add the turkey to a roasting pan.

5. Cover the turkey with the butter.

6. Cover with foil.

7. Add to the grill and cook for another 1 hour.

8. Let rest for 20 minutes before carving and serving.

Nutrition:

- Calories 935
- Total fat 53g
- Saturated fat 15g
- Protein 107g
- Sodium 320mg

37. Traeger Grilled Chicken

Preparation Time: 10 Minutes
Cooking Time: 1 Hour and 10 Minutes
Servings: 6
Ingredients:

- 5 lb. whole chicken

- 1/2 cup oil

- Traeger chicken rub

Directions:

1. Preheat the Traeger on the smoke setting with the lid open for 5 minutes. Close the lid, and let it warm for 15 minutes or until it reaches 450.

2. Use bakers' twine to tie the chicken legs together, then rub it with oil. Coat the chicken with the rub and place it on the grill.

3. Grill for 70 minutes with the lid closed or until it reaches an internal temperature of 1650F.

4. Remove the chicken from the Traeger and let rest for 15 minutes. Cut and serve.

Nutrition:

- Calories 935
- Total fat 53g
- Saturated fat 15g
- Protein 107g
- Sodium 320mg

38. Traeger Chicken Breast

Preparation Time: 10 Minutes
Cooking Time: 15 Minutes
Servings: 6
Ingredients:

- Three chicken breasts

- 1 tbsp avocado oil

- 1/4 tbsp garlic powder

- 1/4 tbsp onion powder

- 3/4 tbsp salt

- 1/4 tbsp pepper

Directions:

1. Preheat your Traeger to 3750F

2. Cut the chicken breast into halves lengthwise, then coat with avocado oil.

3. Season with garlic powder, onion powder, salt, and pepper.

4. Place the chicken on the grill and cook for 7 minutes on each side or until the internal temperature reaches 1650F

Nutrition:

- Calories 120
- Total fat 4g
- Saturated fat 1g
- Protein 19g

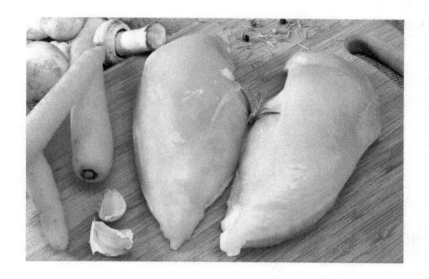

39. Trager Smoked Spatchcock Turkey

Preparation Time: 30 Minutes
Cooking Time: 1 Hour and 15 Minutes
Servings: 8
Ingredients:

- One turkey

- 1/2 cup melted butter

- 1/4 cup Traeger chicken rub

- 1 tbsp onion powder

- 1 tbsp garlic powder

- 1 tbsp rubbed sage

Directions:

1. Preheat your Traeger to high temperature.

2. Put the turkey on a chopping board with the breast side down and the legs pointing towards you.

3. Cut either side of the turkey backbone to remove the spine. Flip the turkey and place it on a pan

4. Season both sides with the seasonings and place it on the grill skin side up on the grill.

5. Cook for 30 minutes, reduce temperature and cook for 45 more minutes until the internal temperature reaches 1650F.

6. Remove from the Traeger and let rest for 15 minutes before slicing and serving.

Nutrition:

- Calories 156
- Total fat 16g
- Saturated fat 2g
- Total carbs 1g
- Net carbs 1g

Fish Recipes

40. Traeger Salmon with Togarashi

Preparation Time: 5 Minutes
Cooking Time: 20 Minutes
Servings: 3
Ingredients:

- One salmon fillet

- 1/4 cup olive oil

- 1/2 tbsp kosher salt

- 1 tbsp Togarashi seasoning

Directions:

1. Preheat your Traeger to 4000F.

2. Place the salmon on a sheet lined with non-stick foil with the skin side down.

3. Rub the oil into the meat, then sprinkle salt and Togarashi.

4. Place the salmon on the grill and cook for 20 minutes or until the internal temperature reaches 1450F with the lid closed.

5. Remove from the Traeger and serve when hot.

Nutrition:

- Calories 119
- Total fat 10g
- Saturated fat 2g
- Sodium 720mg

41. Trager Rockfish

Preparation Time: 10 Minutes
Cooking Time: 20 Minutes
Servings: 6
Ingredients:

- Six rockfish fillets

- One lemon, sliced

- 3/4 tbsp salt

- 2 tbsp fresh dill, chopped

- 1/2 tbsp garlic powder

- 1/2 tbsp onion powder

- 6 tbsp butter

Directions:

1. Preheat your Traeger to 4000F.

2. Season the fish with salt, dill, garlic, and onion powder on both sides, then place it in a baking dish.

3. Place a pat of butter and a lemon slice on each fillet. Place the baking dish in the Traeger and close the lid.

4. Cook for 20 minutes or until the fish is no longer translucent and is flaky.

5. Remove from Traeger and let rest before serving.

Nutrition:

- Calories 270
- Total fat 17g
- Saturated fat 9g

- Total carbs 2g
- Net carbs 2g
- Protein 28g
- Sodium 381mg

42. Traeger Grilled Lingcod

Preparation Time: 10 Minutes
Cooking Time: 15 Minutes
Servings: 6
Ingredients:

- 2 lb. lingcod fillets

- 1/2 tbsp salt

- 1/2 tbsp white pepper

- 1/4 tbsp cayenne pepper

- Lemon wedges

Directions:

1. Preheat your Traeger to 3750F.

2. Place the lingcod on a parchment paper or a grill mat

3. Season the fish with salt, pepper, and top with lemon wedges.

4. Cook the fish for 15 minutes or until the internal temperature reaches 1450F.

Nutrition:

- Calories 245
- Total fat 2g
- Total carbs 2g
- Protein 52g
- Sugars 1g
- Fiber 1g
- Sodium 442mg

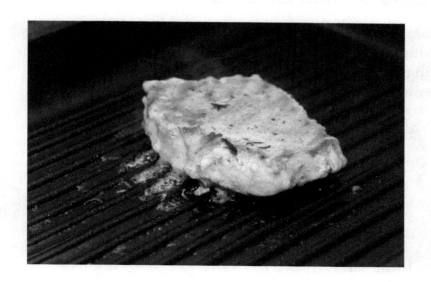

43. Crab Stuffed Lingcod

Preparation Time: 20 Minutes
Cooking Time: 30 Minutes
Servings: 6
Ingredients:
Lemon cream sauce

- Four garlic cloves

- One shallot

- One leek

- 2 tbsp olive oil

- 1 tbsp salt

- 1/4 tbsp black pepper

- 3 tbsp butter

- 1/4 cup white wine

- 1 cup whipping cream

- 2 tbsp lemon juice

- 1 tbsp lemon zest

Crab mix

- 1 lb. crab meat

- 1/3 cup mayo

- 1/3 cup sour cream

- 1/3 cup lemon cream sauce

- 1/4 green onion, chopped

- 1/4 tbsp black pepper

- 1/2 tbsp old bay seasoning

Fish

- 2 lb. lingcod

- 1 tbsp olive oil

- 1 tbsp salt

- 1 tbsp paprika

- 1 tbsp green onion, chopped

- 1 tbsp Italian parsley

Directions:

Lemon cream sauce

1. Chop garlic, shallot, and leeks, then add to a saucepan with oil, salt, pepper, and butter.

2. Sauté over medium heat until the shallot is translucent.

3. Deglaze with white wine, then add whipping cream. Bring the sauce to boil, reduce heat, and simmer for 3 minutes.

4. Remove from heat and add lemon juice and lemon zest. Transfer the sauce to a blender and blend until smooth.

5. Set aside 1/3 cup for the crab mix

Crab mix

1. Add all the fixings to a mixing bowl and mix thoroughly until well combined.

2. Set aside

Fish

1. Fire up your Traeger to high heat, then slice the fish into 6-ounce portions.

2. Lay the fish on its side on a cutting board and slice it 3/4 way through the middle leaving a 1/2 inch on each end to have a nice pouch.

3. Rub the oil into the fish, then place them on a baking sheet. Sprinkle with salt.

4. Stuff crab mix into each fish, then sprinkle paprika and place it on the grill.

5. Cook for 15 minutes or more if the fillets are more than 2 inches thick.

6. Remove the fish and transfer to serving platters. Pour the remaining lemon cream sauce on each fish and garnish with onions and parsley.

Nutrition:

- Calories 476
- Total fat 33g
- Saturated fat 14g
- Total carbs 6g
- Net carbs 5g
- Protein 38g
- Sugars 3g
- Fiber 1g
- Sodium 1032mg

44. Traeger Smoked Shrimp

Preparation Time: 10 Minutes
Cooking Time: 10 Minutes
Servings: 6
Ingredients:

- 1 lb. tail-on shrimp, uncooked

- 1/2 tbsp onion powder

- 1/2 tbsp garlic powder

- 1/2 tbsp salt

- 4 tbsp teriyaki sauce

- 2 tbsp green onion, minced

- 4 tbsp sriracha mayo

Directions:

1. Peel the shrimp shells leaving the tail on, then wash well and rise.

2. Drain well and pat dry with a paper towel.

3. Preheat your Traeger to 4500F.

4. Season the shrimp with onion powder, garlic powder, and salt. Place the shrimp in the Traeger and cook for 6 minutes on each side.

5. Remove the shrimp from the Traeger and toss with teriyaki sauce, then garnish with onions and mayo.

Nutrition:

- Calories 87
- Total carbs 2g

- Net carbs 2g
- Protein 16g
- Sodium 1241mg

45. Grilled Shrimp Kabobs

Preparation Time: 5 Minutes
Cooking Time: 10 Minutes
Servings: 4
Ingredients:

- 1 lb. colossal shrimp, peeled and deveined

- 2 tbsp. oil

- 1/2 tbsp. garlic salt

- 1/2 tbsp. salt

- 1/8 tbsp. pepper

- Six skewers

Directions:

1. Preheat your Traeger to 3750F.

2. Pat the shrimp dry with a paper towel.

3. In a mixing bowl, mix oil, garlic salt, salt, and pepper

4. Toss the shrimp in the mixture until well coated.

5. Skewer the shrimps and cook in the Traeger with the lid closed for 4 minutes.

6. Open the lid, flip the skewers, cook for another 4 minutes, or wait until the shrimp is pink and the flesh is opaque.

7. Serve.

Nutrition:

- Calories 325

- Protein 20g
- Sodium 120mg

46. Bacon-Wrapped Shrimp

Preparation Time: 20 Minutes
Cooking Time: 10 Minutes
Servings: 12
Ingredients:

- 1 lb. raw shrimp

- 1/2 tbsp salt

- 1/4 tbsp garlic powder

- 1 lb. bacon, cut into halves

Directions:

1. Preheat your Traeger to 3500F.

2. Remove the shells and tails from the shrimp, then pat them dry with the paper towels.

3. Sprinkle salt and garlic on the shrimp, then wrap with bacon and secure with a toothpick.

4. Place the shrimps on a baking rack greased with cooking spray.

5. Cook for 10 minutes, flip and cook for another 10 minutes, or until the bacon is crisp enough.

6. Remove from the Traeger and serve.

Nutrition:

- Calories 204
- Total fat 14g
- Saturated fat 5g
- Total carbs 1g
- Net carbs 1g

- Protein 18g
- Sodium 939mg

47. Traeger Spot Prawn Skewers

Preparation Time: 10 Minutes
Cooking Time: 10 Minutes
Servings: 6
Ingredients:

- 2 lb. spot prawns

- 2 tbsp oil

- Salt and pepper to taste

Directions:

1. Preheat your Traeger to 4000F.

2. Skewer your prawns with soaked skewers, then generously sprinkle with oil, salt, and pepper.

3. Place the skewers on the grill, then cook with the lid closed for 5 minutes on each side.

4. Remove the skewers and serve when hot.

Nutrition:

- Calories 221
- Total fat 7g
- Saturated fat 1g
- Total carbs 2g
- Net carbs 2g
- Protein 34g
- Sodium 1481mg

48. Traeger Bacon-wrapped Scallops

Preparation Time: 15 Minutes
Cooking Time: 20 Minutes
Servings: 8
Ingredients:

- 1 lb. sea scallops

- 1/2 lb. bacon

- Sea salt

Directions:

1. Preheat your Traeger to 3750F.

2. Pat dry the scallops with a towel, then wrap them with a piece of bacon and secure with a toothpick.

3. Lay the scallops on the grill with the bacon side down. Close the lid and cook for 5 minutes on each side.

4. Keep the scallops on the bacon side so that you will not get grill marks on the scallops.

5. Serve and enjoy.

Nutrition:

- Calories 261
- Total fat 14g
- Saturated fat 5g
- Total carbs 5g
- Net carbs 5g
- Protein 28g
- Sodium 1238mg

49. Traeger Lobster Tail

Preparation Time: 10 Minutes
Cooking Time: 15 Minutes
Servings: 2
Ingredients:

- 10 oz lobster tail

- 1/4 tbsp old bay seasoning

- 1/4 tbsp Himalayan salt

- 2 tbsp butter, melted

- 1 tbsp fresh parsley, chopped

Directions:

1. Preheat your Traeger to 4500F.

2. Slice the tail down the middle, then season it with bay seasoning and salt.

3. Place the tails directly on the grill with the meat side down. Grill for 15 minutes or until the internal temperature reaches 1400F.

4. Remove from the Traeger and drizzle with butter.

5. Serve when hot garnished with parsley.

Nutrition:

- Calories 305
- Total fat 14g
- Saturated fat 8g
- Total carbs 5g
- Net carbs 5g
- Protein 38g

- Sodium 684mg

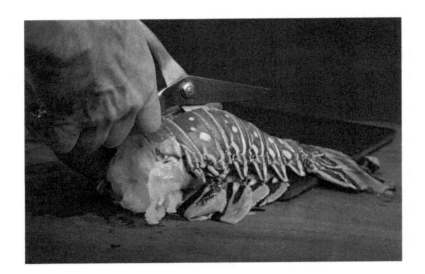

50. Roasted Honey Salmon

Preparation Time: 5 Minutes
Cooking Time: 1 Hour
Servings: 4
Ingredients:

- Two cloves garlic, grated

- Two tablespoon ginger, minced

- One teaspoon honey

- One teaspoon sesame oil

- Two tablespoon lemon juice

- One teaspoon chili paste

- Four salmon fillets

- Two tablespoon soy sauce

Directions:

1. Set your wood pellet grill to smoke while the lid is open.

2. Do this for 5 minutes.

3. Preheat your wood pellet grill to 400 degrees F.

4. Combine all the ingredients except salmon in a sealable plastic bag.

5. Shake to mix the ingredients.

6. Add the salmon.

7. Marinate inside the refrigerator for 30 minutes.

8. Add the salmon to a roasting pan and place it on top of the grill.

9. Close the lid and cook for 3 minutes.

10. Flip the salmon and cook for another 3 minutes.

Nutrition:

- Calories 119
- Total fat 10g
- Saturated fat 2g
- Sodium 720mg

51. Blackened Salmon

Preparation Time: 10 Minutes
Cooking Time: 20 Minutes
Servings: 4
Ingredients:

- 2 lb. salmon, fillet, scaled and deboned

- Two tablespoons olive oil

- Four tablespoons sweet dry rub

- One tablespoon cayenne pepper

- Two cloves garlic, minced

Directions:

1. Turn on your wood pellet grill.

2. Set it to 350 degrees F.

3. Brush the salmon with the olive oil.

4. Sprinkle it with the dry rub, cayenne pepper, and garlic.

5. Grill for 5 minutes per side.

Nutrition:

- Calories 119
- Total fat 10g
- Saturated fat 2g
- Sodium 720mg

52. Grilled Cajun Shrimp

Preparation Time: 5 Minutes
Cooking Time: 25 Minutes
Servings: 8
Ingredients:
Dip

- 1/2 cup mayonnaise

- One teaspoon lemon juice

- 1 cup sour cream

- One clove garlic, grated

- One tablespoon Cajun seasoning

- One tablespoon hickory bacon rub

- One tablespoon hot sauce

- Chopped scallions

Shrimp

- 1/2 lb. shrimp, peeled and deveined

- Two tablespoons olive oil

- 1/2 tablespoon hickory bacon seasoning

- One tablespoon Cajun seasoning

Directions:

1. Turn on your wood pellet grill.

2. Set it to 350 degrees F.

3. Mix the dip ingredients in a bowl.

4. Transfer to a small pan.

5. Cover with foil.

6. Place on top of the grill.

7. Cook for 10 minutes.

8. Coat the shrimp with the olive oil and sprinkle with the seasonings.

9. Grill for 5 minutes per side.

10. Pour the dip on top or serve with the shrimp.

Nutrition:

- Calories 87
- Total carbs 2g
- Net carbs 2g
- Protein 16g
- Sodium 1241mg

53. Salmon Cakes

Preparation Time: 5 Minutes
Cooking Time: 25 Minutes
Servings: 4
Ingredients:

- 1 cup cooked salmon, flaked

- 1/2 red bell pepper, chopped

- Two eggs, beaten

- 1/4 cup mayonnaise

- 1/2 tablespoon dry sweet rub

- 1 1/2 cups breadcrumbs

- One tablespoon mustard

- Olive oil

Directions:

1. Combine all the fixings except the olive oil in a bowl.

2. Form patties from this mixture.

3. Let sit for 15 minutes.

4. Turn on your wood pellet grill.

5. Set it to 350 degrees F.

6. Add a baking pan to the grill.

7. Drizzle a little olive oil on top of the pan.

8. Add the salmon cakes to the pan.

9. Grill each side for 3 to 4 minutes.

Nutrition:

- Calories 119
- Total fat 10g
- Saturated fat 2g
- Sodium 720mg

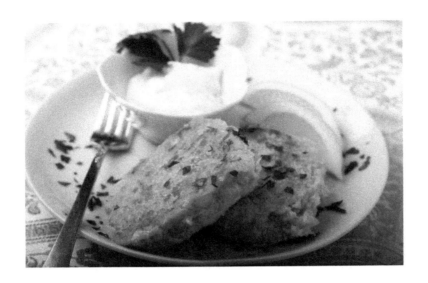

CPSIA information can be obtained
at www.ICGtesting.com
Printed in the USA
BVHW062105250221
601128BV00006BA/453